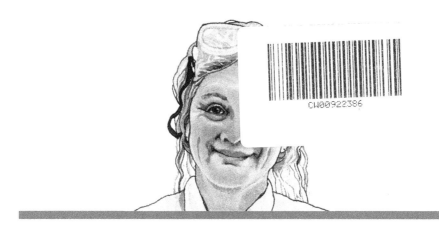

Cool Soapmaking
The Smart Guide to
Low-Temp Tricks for Making Soap

— Anne L. Watson —

Soapmakers may love to add a variety of materials to soap, but they find that some cause more trouble than others. In the heat of the chemical reaction, an ingredient might discolor, or lose its scent, or develop a bad smell. Or it might cause problems during soapmaking, giving off noxious fumes, or making the soap harden so fast that there's no time to pour it in the mold.

Help has arrived.

Anne L. Watson extends the low-temp techniques from her book *Milk Soapmaking* to making soap from a variety of special ingredients, including cucumber, citrus, pine tar, beer, and wine. Soaps that have long challenged home soapmakers will now pose no problem at all.

BOOKS BY ANNE L. WATSON

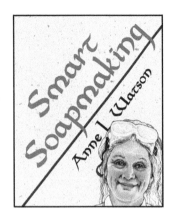
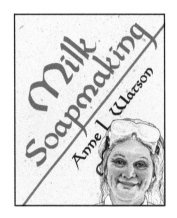
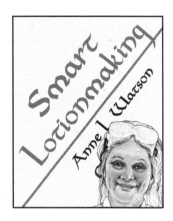
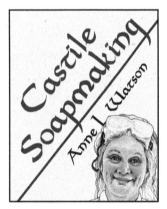
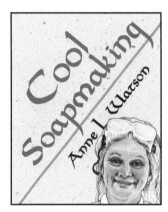
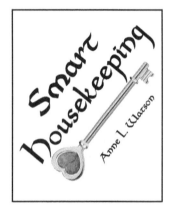
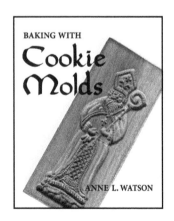
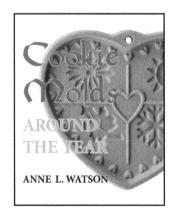
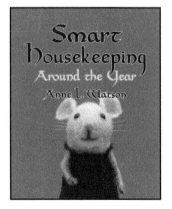

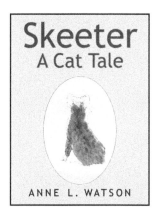

Skeeter
A Cat Tale
ANNE L. WATSON

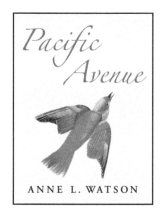

Pacific
Avenue
ANNE L. WATSON

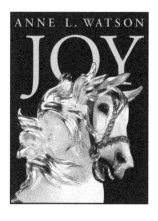

ANNE L. WATSON
JOY

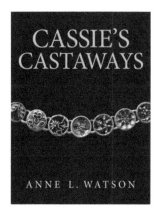

CASSIE'S
CASTAWAYS
ANNE L. WATSON

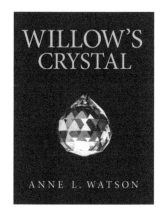

WILLOW'S
CRYSTAL
ANNE L. WATSON

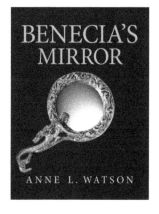

BENECIA'S
MIRROR
ANNE L. WATSON

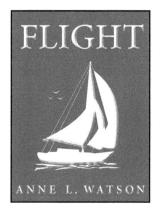

FLIGHT
ANNE L. WATSON

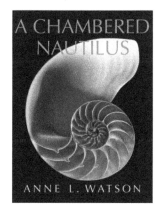

A CHAMBERED
NAUTILUS
ANNE L. WATSON

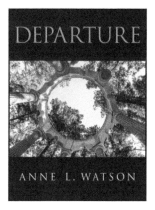

DEPARTURE
ANNE L. WATSON

and more . . .

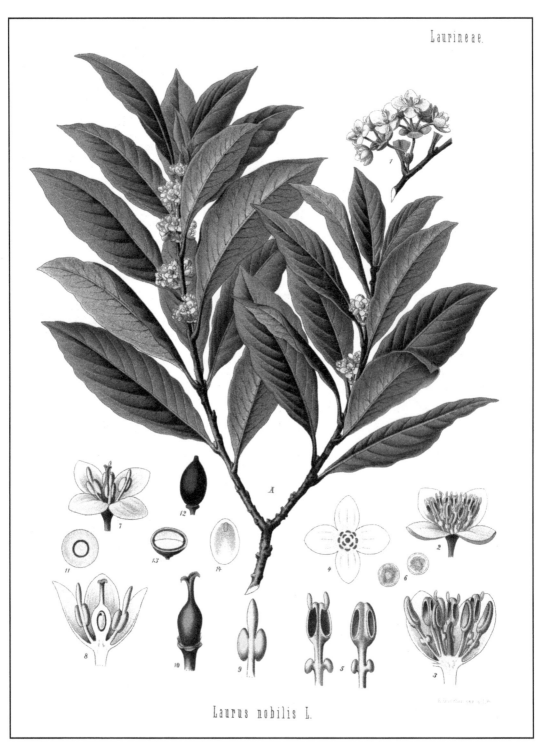

"Laurus nobilis L."—old botanical print of sweet bay

Cool Soapmaking

The Smart Guide to
Low-Temp Tricks for Making Soap

OR

How to Handle Fussy Ingredients
Like Milk, Citrus, Cucumber,
Pine Tar, Beer, and Wine

Anne L. Watson

Shepard Publications
Bellingham, Washington

Special thanks to Susan Kennedy of Oregon Trail Soaps for my
introduction to low-temp soapmaking.

Version 1.2

Contents

Getting Started
From High-Temp Soapmaking to Low

From the beginning of soapmaking, people have made it "hot." In fact, professional soapmakers used to be called soap boilers and shared a patron saint with firefighters.

As far as I can tell, the kind of soapmaking now called *hot process* was the rule for both family and commercial soapmaking all the way up to around 1940. At that time, companies that manufactured lye began to market it for home soapmaking, which was falling out of fashion. The new method came to be known as *cold process*—a term I've found from as early as that same period, in a lye company pamphlet.

Though in cold process the soap mixture isn't "cooked," it isn't really cold either, as its temperature usually falls somewhere between room temperature and 110°F (43°C). Still, cold process seemed simpler, possibly safer, and was less intimidating to beginners. So, as craft soapmaking became popular, cold process was the technique favored in many books.

More recently, soapmakers adding milk to their soaps have come up with a version of cold process that truly does involve lower temperatures. In my book *Milk Soapmaking*, I called it Cool Technique. It uses frozen liquid to counteract the heat generated by the dissolving lye. This aims to keep the milk as cold as possible, to avoid browning the milk sugars and darkening the soap.

After writing that book, I continued to refine Cool Technique. But more important, I discovered that its usefulness goes far beyond milk soap. In fact, it can help wherever high temperatures cause problems of scorching, fumes, acceleration, or other unwanted reactions. And that's very cool!

IMPORTANT!

Since low-temp soapmaking is a specialty, this book assumes you already have some experience in craft soapmaking. If that's not true, please set this one aside for a while and read my book *Smart Soapmaking*, or at least *Milk Soapmaking*. That will give you the background you need to make soap and do it safely.

What Do I Put Into It?
The Ingredients of Cool Soapmaking

Since you can use Cool Technique with any recipe, it doesn't in itself require much in the way of special ingredients. Of course, as we discuss the kinds of soaps it's good for, I'll say what you need for each kind.

Please note that Cool Technique recipes include liquid ingredients that must be prepared in advance, and some have other ingredients to prepare as well. Also, some recipes ask you to set aside part of the base fats to mix with another ingredient.

For low-temp soapmaking, I generally recommend microbead lye, also called food-grade lye. (Yes, lye is used in some commercial food preparation.) This type is best because it dissolves quickly in cold liquid. But I don't recommend it for real beginners, because it's very light and scatters easily.

If you don't use microbead lye, use bead lye. Never use flake lye with Cool Technique.

What Do I Use to Make It?
Gathering the Equipment You Need

Your choice of soap mold is important in Cool Technique. For most projects, tray molds or individual molds are best because they cool quickest. Use molds made of materials that transmit heat fairly quickly—silicone is good, wood not as much. For projects with trace accelerants, though, you need a log mold with a smooth surface, as explained in that chapter.

Here are a few more special items you'll need.

• Tray for supporting your soap molds, if they're silicone.
• Plastic wrap, to cover the soap in the mold and discourage soda ash.
• Ice cube trays, two or more. I strongly prefer the ones that make tiny cubes, about a quarter inch on a side. When mixed with lye, these small cubes are much less likely to cause splashing than are larger cubes or irregularly shaped bits of ice.

The rest of what you need is pretty much the same as for general soapmaking.

• Safety equipment—gloves, goggles, apron, and solid shoes.
• Digital scale, weighing grams or tenths of an ounce.
• Thermometer—waterproof, "instant-read," digital.
• Soup pot or other large pot.
• Saucepan.
• Microwave-safe bowl or glass measuring pitcher for solid fat.
• Bowl or glass measuring cup for weighing lye.

• Container for weighing liquid fats. (But forget this if there's only one kind of liquid fat in the recipe. In that case, you'll weigh it in the soup pot.)

• Containers for weighing scent and colorant (if you're using them).

• Stick blender.

• Long-handled spoon—steel, stainless steel, or plastic.

• Spatula—rubber or silicone. At least one, preferably two.

• Sieve.

• pH papers that read at least between the values of 7 and 14. (Highly recommended).

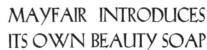

MAYFAIR INTRODUCES ITS OWN BEAUTY SOAP

by John Dew of Bond Street.

Yesterday, Milady had no soap equal in breeding to her gowns, shoes and perfume. To-day, John Dew of Mayfair is making a soap, costly, it is true, but enfolding a beauty secret for which Society would have been willing to barter its jewels.

The name, John Dew's Milk Soap, reveals the secret. In it lies all the loveliness that famous beauties of long ago found by bathing in milk. Its creamy lather is gentle as a caress to the most fragile complexion; its fragrance, delicate and evanescent, retreats before the individuality of one's chosen perfume.

★ ★ ★

Sold by all high class chemists and stores. 1/= a tablet, 3/= per box of 3 tablets.

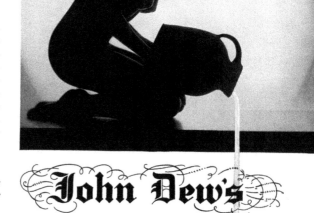

Prepared under Exclusive
Proprietary Process by

John Dew.

JOHN DEW LTD.,
180, NEW BOND ST.,
LONDON, W.1.

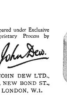

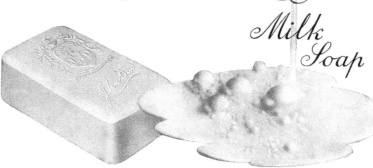

Ad for John Dew's Milk Soap, 1932

Project #1
Milk Soaps

I've tried making soaps with most popular kinds of animal milk, and with many kinds of vegetable milk as well. I think they all make good soap. Fat content matters to some extent, of course. But I doubt I could tell cow milk soap from goat.

There are many legends about bathing in milk—even Cleopatra is said to have done it. The earliest advertisement I've found for milk soap is from 1932. Whether its claims are accurate, I don't know, but the ad says the soap in question is a revival of an ancient beauty secret.

Why use Cool Technique for milk soap? Many soapmakers want their milk soaps to be "milk white." But if milk soaps are made hot or even at room temperature, they will turn out tan or brown. So the main point of low-temp soapmaking for milk soaps is to stabilize the color. (I've read that browning also reduces lather, but I can't say I've tested that.)

Anne's Cool Milk Soap

Here is the recipe I recommend for your first effort at Cool Technique soapmaking. (If it looks familiar, it's the same one I gave in *Milk Soapmaking*.) This can be made with any animal milk, fresh or reconstituted, and with some plant milks.

It's handy to copy this recipe so you don't have to flip pages back and forth as you work through the instructions.

    9 oz (255 g) coconut oil
    21 oz (595 g) olive oil
    9 oz (255 g) fluid milk (cow, goat, coconut, soy, etc.)
    4.1 oz (116 g) lye

**Before proceeding, read the following pages
thoroughly to understand the method!**

Cool Soapmaking Step-by-Step
From Prep to Cleanup and Beyond

Here I'll describe in detail how to make soap with Cool Technique. These sample instructions are for my basic milk soap recipe, but you'll easily be able to adapt them for later recipes. (If you've already read my book *Milk Soapmaking*, this will mostly be just review.)

Don't forget safety. Protect yourself from the slightest contact with the lye or the soap mixture at all times. From the moment you open a container of lye until cleanup is complete, you must wear rubber gloves, goggles, protective clothing, and solid shoes. Watch your hands and your work carefully as you weigh and add the lye. Make sure there is no spillage. If there is, clean it up immediately.

For lye mixing, it's best to work under a range hood with the fan on, and with the lye solution as far away from your face as possible. Some soapmakers work outdoors or near a window—but if you're using microbead lye, either of these locations can be too breezy. You do *not* want your lye to scatter.

Wherever your lye mixing area is, keep other people and pets away from it. If you work on a table that's painted or varnished, protect the surface with a tarp or other waterproof covering.

The Day Before

Weigh the liquid—in this case, the milk—and pour it into an ice cube tray. Put it in the freezer for the next day's soapmaking.

Preparing Ingredients

1. Weigh the liquid fat—in this case, the olive oil—in your soapmaking pot.

2. Weigh the solid fat—in this case, the coconut oil—in the large microwave-safe bowl or pitcher.

3. Heat the solid fat in your microwave till it is barely melted. The exact time needed depends on the quantity and type of solid fat and also on your microwave. If you catch it while there are a few solid bits left, that's ideal. Remove it from the microwave and stir until everything is melted.

4. Add the melted fat to the liquid fat in the soapmaking pot.

5. Take your cubes of pre-weighed frozen milk from the freezer and put them in your saucepan.

Mixing the Lye Solution

1. PUT ON YOUR GOGGLES AND GLOVES.

2. Make sure your bowl or glass cup for measuring lye is completely dry and free of any fats, as is anything else that might contact the lye.

3. Weigh the lye for your recipe in the bowl or cup. Note: In rare cases, static electricity will make the lye grains scatter as they're poured. This is more likely to happen with microbead lye than with bead lye. If you see this happen, spoon out the lye instead of pouring it. (You can also get rid of the static electricity ahead of time by wiping the bowl or cup with a dryer sheet.)

4. Add the lye to the frozen milk cubes in the saucepan, stirring carefully with the long-handled, slotted spoon. Note that a mixture of ice and liquid is *more* likely to splash than liquid alone would be. So, be sure to keep the pot at arm's length while you stir, and stir carefully.

As the lye dissolves, the ice cubes will melt. Working cold like this, you'll generally have far less fumes than when you use room temperature liquid. All the same, you need good ventilation.

Another reason to have good ventilation: Lye and milk protein react in a way that produces an ammonia-like smell. It's usually faint and goes away, but avoid breathing much of these fumes. But don't panic either, as many soapmakers do when they smell it. It's normal.

As you mix the milk with the lye, the milk usually changes color, at least a little. Even if it turns really ugly, keep going, because it almost certainly won't stay that way.

Another thing you may see is grainy texture. I've read instructions for milk soapmaking that say you must throw away your lye mixture if this happens—all is lost! That's a myth, though. The graininess is caused by coagulation of proteins in the lye solution. It makes no difference at all, especially if you're using a stick blender. A bit of trivia: This effect will most often be noticed with lower-fat milk.

Yet another effect produced by dissolving lye in milk is that the fat in the milk begins to saponify. If you're using cream, you will get a fairly stiff mixture at this point. Once again, you can find advice to the effect that the soap is worthless if this happens—and once again, it's just not so.

5. With an opaque liquid, you can't tell just by looking if the lye is dissolved.

Luckily, there's a different way you can tell, as provided by a chemist I consulted. Once all the milk is melted, take the temperature of the mixture. At first, the temperature will seesaw or even rise. Stir the mixture a bit and keep checking. When the temperature definitely begins to fall, the lye is dissolved.

I found only one exception to this rule, and that's when you're making soap with high-fat liquids like cream. Because of the high proportion of fat, there's enough saponification that the temperature will continue to rise. In that case, just keep stirring for four or five minutes—that should be enough.

Not sure whether the amount of fat in your mixture will keep the temperature rising or let it fall? Here's an easy way to tell: If there's enough to keep the temperature rising, the mixture will also thicken noticeably as you stir. As long as it stays thin, you can count on a temperature drop to tell you the lye is dissolved.

Combining the Ingredients

1. Pour the milk-and-lye solution through the sieve and into the soap pot with the fat. Or, if it's too thick to pour—as it will be with recipes that use high-fat milks—press it through the sieve with a rubber spatula.

2. Stir with the long-handled spoon until mixed. Don't worry if the soap still has an ammonia-like smell. It will go away. But you should use good ventilation and avoid breathing the fumes.

3. Add any scent or liquid colorant and stir it in a bit.

4. Maintaining good ventilation, mix with the stick blender. Move it throughout the mixture so everything gets blended thoroughly, tipping the pot as you need to. While the stick blender is running, be careful to keep the blade submerged, or you'll stir air into the soap and may splash the mixture. Whenever you lift the blade out, take your finger off the button so the blade stops spinning before reaching the surface.

Keep blending the mixture, and you'll begin to see changes. Originally oily and transparent, it will become creamy and opaque. The surface, which was shiny at first, will become duller, and the oily ring at the edge of the mixture's surface—right where it meets the wall of the pot—will shrink and all but disappear.

Next you'll notice the mixture thickening and getting smoother. It will come to resemble thick eggnog or very thin pudding. At this point, you can stop blending, because the saponification that produces soap can continue without further mixing. You might call this "the point of no return."

Besides the visual signs, you can get a feel for the thickening by turning off the blender and briefly stirring with a spoon. With a weaker blender, you can even *hear* the difference, as the thickening slows down the blade, causing the sound of the motor to drop in pitch.

You should have little trouble recognizing the signs I've given— but if you're not sure, leave the stick blender off and hand-stir with it for about thirty seconds to see if the mixture thins out again. If it does, go back to blending. Good lighting makes a huge difference with the visual tests.

A special, though rare, consideration: With cold ingredients, you can get obvious thickening as soon as you start blending, most likely from the melted fat resolidifying as it blends with the cool lye solution. This is actually "false trace," and the way to deal with it is to stir with your spoon until the soap thins again. But some soaps actually are ready to pour in a minute or two. One way to tell is with a thermometer. With false trace, you won't see a temperature rise.

Molding

1. Pour the mixture into your mold, scraping the pot with the rubber spatula. If your mold is flexible, make sure it sits on a rack or other rigid support you can use to move it. Never move a flexible mold full of unhardened soap mixture by itself!

2. When the soap has set a bit, cover it with plastic wrap. This will almost always prevent soda ash, a powdery residue that can be a special problem with low-temp soapmaking. You want the wrap to shut out as much air as possible, so don't let it

wrinkle. On the other hand, don't push the wrap into the soap face so it sticks!

3. Put the mold in the refrigerator for at least three hours. Or if you want the palest possible color, first set it in the freezer for half an hour, then move it to the refrigerator. Just don't forget to take it out of the freezer!

Later, when you take the mold from the refrigerator, you can set it on a counter or other location at room temperature.

Removal and Testing

Your soap should be solid in about twelve hours, and ready to come out of the mold and be tested in about twenty-four. At this point, the soap shouldn't be caustic, but you should work with your gloves on till you test it and you're sure.

Put a little distilled water on the surface of the soap, scrub a bit to make a paste, then push a pH strip into the paste. If the strip shows anything in the range of 7 to 10, the soap is fine. The exact pH reading doesn't matter—the strips don't measure all that accurately anyway. But they *will* let you know if your soap is in a safe range.

If the pH strip reads 11 or 12, let the soap sit for a few days and test it again. It may just need a little more time. If your reading is above 12, don't use the soap and don't even touch it without gloves. Sometimes a very high pH will slowly decrease till the soap is usable. More often, the soap should be discarded or rebatched.

If the outer surface tests OK, slice the block in half and look at the cut surfaces. Your soap should have a texture that's fairly smooth and regular, with a consistency like cheese. It may be slightly sticky on the cut edges, and there may be a small difference in texture or color between the cut faces and the outer surface of the block—something like a rind covering a soft cheese. This is normal.

Test one of the cut surfaces with a pH strip. Also test anything that looks unusual—a shiny patch, a light spot, anything that stands out from the rest. Once in a long while, you may get a high reading on something that looks "off." When that happens to me, I discard or rebatch the entire block.

If it all tests OK, you're home free.

Cutting and Curing

After testing out successfully, your soap is ready to cut into bars, if you need to do that. But cutting milk soap can be tricky. It may tend to chip, especially at the bottom of the cut. Sometimes, waiting another day will solve the problem. But sometimes it won't.

One simple solution is to turn your slab of soap on edge to cut it. Another is to use a large, sharp pizza-cutting wheel. Yet another, mostly for shorter cuts, is to use a cheese wire.

Soap should dry out for a while, which also gives it a chance to grow milder. Set the bars somewhere with good air circulation, on a rack if possible. Curing time depends on how much liquid went into the soap, as well as on how it's stored and how humid the storage area. Minimum times normally range from a couple of weeks to a month, with the time for soaps from most of my recipes falling about halfway between, at three weeks. Soap with a very high percentage of liquid fat may need to dry even longer than a month.

How can you be sure the soap is dry enough? Just try a bar. If the lather is stringy or slimy, or if the soap gets used up too fast or gets gooey, that soap needs more time. The longer the bars dry—up to a couple of months or so—the harder they'll become and the longer they'll last in use.

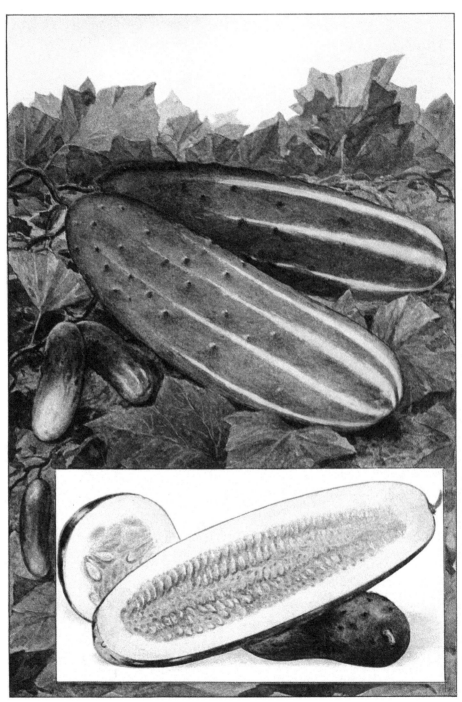

"Cucumbers"—old botanical print

Project #2
Cucumber Soaps

According to *The Cambridge World History of Food*, cucumbers have been used in soaps and other cosmetics since at least the 1800s. Many people have loved cucumber soap.

Some of the claims made for this soap are a little confusing. It's supposed to be good for acne, but also for dryness and aging skin. And besides soothing the skin and improving the complexion, it's supposed to make freckles fade. Occasionally it's even said to cure more serious skin conditions—but as soapmakers, we know we can't legally make such claims.

In any case, cucumbers do make a pleasant soap—slightly astringent and not particularly emollient. The flecks of peel are slightly exfoliating—not as much as cornmeal or coffee grounds would be, but noticeably a little rough. Some believe that cucumber juice is an accelerant, but in my experiments, it wasn't.

Why use Cool Technique for cucumber soaps? As I looked at comments on cucumber soap recipes online, I saw one that occurred over and over: The lye burns the cucumber, producing a nasty odor. Some say the odor fades, others say it doesn't.

I started wondering if it would help to treat cucumber—and possibly other fruit and vegetable soaps as well—the same way we treat milk soaps. In other words, could I avoid burning by freezing the liquid in ice cube trays and sprinkling the lye onto the cucumber "ice cubes"?

It worked perfectly—and not only with cucumber juice or pulp. Since I was freezing the liquid anyway, I found I could even combine the cucumber with a milk product.

Basic Cucumber Soap

21 oz (595 g) olive oil
9 oz (255 g) coconut oil
9 oz (255 g) cucumber juice or puree, frozen
4.3 oz (121 g) lye

Cucumber Yogurt Soap

This recipe makes a nice looking beige soap with green flecks and excellent lather, both bubbly and creamy.

>   21 oz (595 g) olive oil
>   9 oz (255 g) coconut oil
>   4.5 oz (128 g) cucumber juice or puree
>   4.5 oz (128 g) plain whole milk yogurt
>   4.3 oz (121 g) lye

Mix the cucumber juice or puree and yogurt the day before and freeze.

Cucumber Green Clay Soap

Mineral-rich green clay—often called French green clay, as it originally came only from France—is said to have properties highly beneficial to skin. Some green clays will produce green soap, but others make the soap turn out beige. If you need to know which color you'll get, consult the vendor.

    21 oz (595 g) olive oil
    9 oz (255 g) coconut oil
    9 oz (255 g) cucumber juice or puree, frozen
    4.3 oz (121 g) lye
    2 tsp green clay

Add the clay to the fats and stick blend to suspend it just before adding the lye solution.

Cucumber Apricot Soap

15.9 oz (451 g) apricot kernel oil
3 oz (85 g) shea butter
2.1 oz (59 g) castor oil
9 oz (255 g) palm kernel oil flakes
10.6 oz (300 g) cucumber juice, frozen
4.2 oz (119 g) lye

Cucumber Avocado Soap

6 oz (171 g) avocado butter
9 oz (255 g) coconut oil
15 oz (425 g) olive oil
9 oz (255 g) cucumber puree or juice, frozen
4.3 oz (121 g) lye

Designing Cucumber Soaps

Cucumber is over 95% water, so you can consider the entire weight of pureed cucumber to be liquid.

Cucumber juice is slightly acidic, which makes the soap a little softer than it would be if made with pure water. So, I suggest making cucumber soaps with a mix of fats that has at least a medium hardness value, and with superfatting at no more than 5%.

Here are some factors affecting color:

• Color depends partly on temperature. If the soap gets warm while it's setting, it will darken.

• For a pale soap, use light-colored fats.

• Soaps with the vegetable pulp in them will be darker than those with only juice.

• When I used whole unpeeled cucumbers pureed with a stick blender, I got beige soap with green flecks.

• I've gotten pale green soap with whole, unpeeled cucumbers pureed in a food processor with the steel blade.

• For a pale soap with green flecks, I minced the peel separately, used cucumber juice for the liquid, and added the peel just before pouring.

• For the palest soap, juice peeled cucumbers in a vegetable juicer.

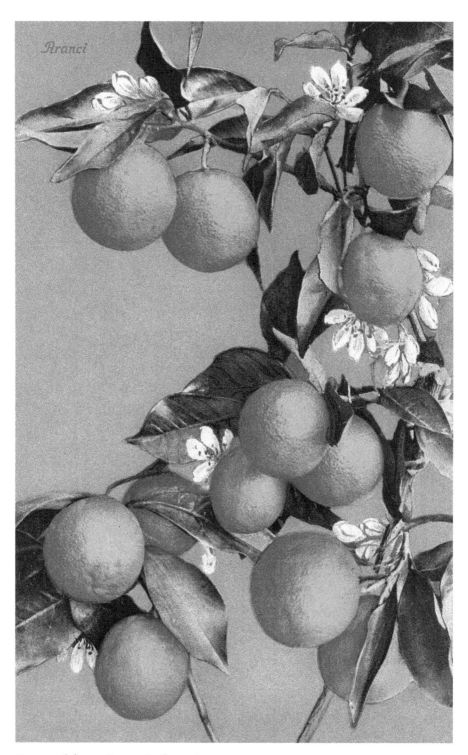

Postcard from Como, Italy, 1932

Project #3
Citrus Soaps

Citrus soaps are popular, and no wonder—they can be lovely. But they can also be disappointing, because the scent is prone to fading.

This is mostly because citrus essential oils are made differently. They are cold-pressed like olive oil, rather than steam-extracted like other essential oils. They just don't fare that well at higher temperatures such as you get in normal soapmaking. But Cool Technique provides better results, giving your soap maximum, lasting aroma.

Some citrus essential oils are concentrated. These are called "five-fold" or "ten-fold" oils (written 5× and 10×). While performing better than other citrus essential oils even in regular soapmaking, the improvement is even more marked with the lower temperatures of Cool Technique.

Some of my recipes combine citrus with milk products. You might wonder if this can cause curdling, but I have yet to see any.

Basic Citrus Soap

12 oz (340 g) coconut oil

6 oz (170 g) olive oil

12 oz (340 g) sunflower oil

9 oz (255 g) water or citrus juice, frozen

4.4 oz (124 g) lye

1.2–2 oz (34–56 g) 10× citrus essential oil, citrus
   fragrance oil, or a blend of scents

Orange Yogurt Soap

This soap was extremely popular with my testers. It has great lather. The peel makes it a scrub soap, so gardeners especially liked it.

> 12 oz (340 g) coconut oil
> 6 oz (170 g) olive oil
> 12 oz (340 g) sunflower oil
> 4.5 oz (128 g) fresh orange juice
> 4.5 oz (128 g) plain whole milk yogurt
> 4.4 oz (124 g) lye
> 1.2–2 oz (34–56 g) 10× citrus essential oil, citrus fragrance oil, or a blend of scents
> 1 tbsp pulverized dried orange peel, soaked in orange essential oil

Mix the juice and yogurt the day before and freeze.

Soak the peel in orange essential oil, preferably 10×, for at least 8 hours before making the soap. Add the peel to the soap along with the scent, just before pouring into the mold.

Citrus Honey Soap

15 oz (425 g) olive oil
9 oz (255 g) coconut oil
6 oz (170 g) walnut oil
7 oz (198 g) half and half (light cream)
2 oz (56 g) orange juice
1 tbsp honey
4.3 oz (121 g) lye
1.2–2 oz (34–56 g) 10× orange essential oil or lemon
    fragrance
1 tbsp pulverized dried lemon or orange peel, soaked in
    lemon essential oil or fragrance oil (optional)

The day before, mix the cream, orange juice, and honey well and freeze the mixture. Expect some acceleration due to the honey.

If using the peel, soak it in essential oil or fragrance oil for at least 8 hours before making the soap. Add the peel to the soap along with the scent, just before pouring into the mold.

Ruby Red Grapefruit Soap

9 oz (255 g) coconut oil
7.5 oz (213 g) avocado oil
3 oz (85 g) sunflower oil
10.5 oz (298 g) olive oil
9 oz (255 g) ruby red grapefruit juice, frozen
4.2 oz (120 g) lye
1.2–2 oz (34–56 g) concentrated grapefruit essential oil,
    or grapefruit fragrance oil
1 tbsp pulverized grapefruit peel, soaked in grapefruit
    essential oil or fragrance oil (optional)

If using the peel, soak it in essential oil or fragrance oil for at least eight hours before making the soap. Add the peel to the soap along with the scent, just before pouring into the mold.

Designing Citrus Soaps

Citrus juices are all more acidic than most soapmaking liquids, which will make for a softer soap. For this reason, consider diluting them with water or milk, and avoid the most acidic citrus juices such as lemon. I recommend a mix of fats with at least a medium hardness value, and superfatting of no more than 5%. Also, the liquid amount should be no more than 30% the weight of the fats.

Some citrus juices and essential oils will color the soap. This might be desirable by itself, but the color of the citrus product will mix with the color of your fats. So, I suggest running small-scale experiments with your intended ingredients to make sure the blended color is attractive. I can imagine a very green olive oil combined with a strongly orange citrus essential oil—you'd probably get gray soap!

For additives, you can make or buy grated, minced, or pulverized citrus peel with many different textures. Again, I recommend small-scale experiments, because you can't always know what an additive will be like in the finished soap. Coarser particles may harden and become too abrasive, while finely pulverized peel may feel gritty or sandy.

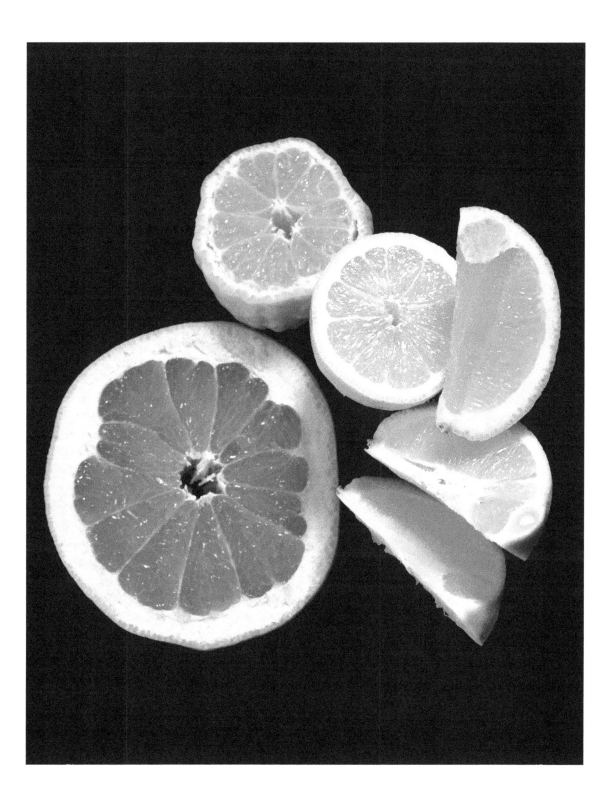

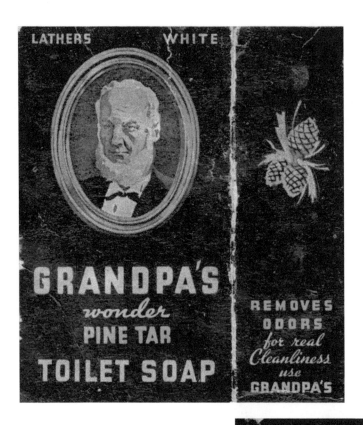

Product box for Grandpa's Wonder Pine Tar Toilet Soap, from The Grandpa Soap Company, Cincinnati

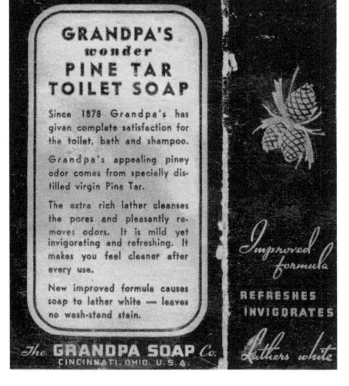

Project #4
Soaps with Accelerants

Certain materials speed up saponification—we generally say they "accelerate trace"— but that's only part of the picture. They speed up everything—saponification, setting, and the rate at which the soap's pH drops to a usable level. In the process, a lot of heat is generated. So, you not only have to avoid the proverbial "soap on a stick"—what you get when the soap thickens too quickly and sets on your spoon. You also need to be concerned about "volcanoes," scorching of fats or other ingredients, and cracking as the soap sets and cures.

To avoid all these, you need to consider both the starting temperatures of your ingredients and how heat can build up after the soap is poured. Yes, the soap in the mold can overheat all on its own, since saponification by itself generates heat. If your molded soap shows signs of overheating, put it in the refrigerator for an hour or so. I have also had good results from placing an overheating silicone mold into a shallow pan of cold water—but if you do this, keep the water from the pan out of your soap!

Accelerants vary in the strength of their effect. The effect of some, like sugar and honey, can be fairly mild, if you don't use too much. Some fragrances and essential oils accelerate quite a bit more—and this can vary from batch to batch of the same oil. Shea oil accelerates quite a bit, as does castor oil. And one notorious accelerant is pine tar.

Cool Technique can help you succeed with any accelerant, as the chemical reaction will be slowed by the lower temperature. It may still be faster than normal, but it will be more manageable.

For the fastest accelerants, though, I've found another trick helpful as well. To make sure my soap doesn't solidify in the pot, I leave out the accelerant while I'm stick blending. Then just as the soap starts to thicken, I pour it into a block or log mold. Only then do I add the accelerant, diluted with a small amount of the base fats I've held back. Finally, I hand stir the rest of the way, being careful to reach into the edges and corners of the mold and all the way to the bottom. This approach can be adapted to any accelerating essential oil, fragrance oil, base oil, or additive.

If your accelerant turns out not as strong as you expected, you may find that the soap does not thicken further with this hand stirring in the mold. In that case, you can switch to your stick blender, being carefully not to splash.

To avoid heat buildup, use molds made of materials that transfer heat quickly. Silicone and plastic are good. Wood not so much, as it retains heat. Also, for hand stirring, it's important that the mold be smooth, as texture or patterns can cause uneven mixing during fast saponification.

With accelerants, I generally use block or log molds even though they do build up more heat, because they allow this hand stirring. But even apart from that, they'd be better than individual molds, because with those, your soap might set before you have time to fill them all. In some cases, the best choice might be a tray mold with dividers. Either way, make sure your mold isn't filled too high, so you don't spill as you're mixing.

Of course, you won't want to insulate your mold! And if you're using more than one, don't place them too close together. That can cause the heat to build till you get a "volcano."

Sweet Bay Soap

I love bay leaves in food and bay essential oil in soap. But the oil is a fierce accelerant and takes almost every trick I know when added to soap. Only a real favorite would be worth so much trouble.

    8 oz (226 g) shea butter
    10 oz (284 g) coconut oil
    12 oz (340 g) grapeseed oil
    11.4 oz (323 g) water, frozen
    4.1 oz (115 g) lye
    1.2–2 oz (34–56 g) bay essential oil

Melt the shea butter and coconut oil together and combine with the grapeseed oil in your soapmaking pot. Let the mixture cool somewhat, but don't let it start to resolidify. Remove one tablespoon of the fats to a small bowl and mix with the bay essential oil.

Prepare the lye solution as usual and add to the soapmaking pot. Stick blend briefly, only to lightly mix the ingredients.

Pour into the log mold and add the bay essential oil mixture. Hand stir with a rubber or silicone spatula, being careful to get into corners and edges.

Pine Tar Soap

Pine tar soap has been made for over a century and is still commercially available today. It is said to be effective for some skin ailments, though the U.S. Food and Drug Administration does not accept it as medically effective. The soap is brown, but the lather is white.

I often get recipe requests for this soap. The problem for soapmakers has been that pine tar is such a strong accelerant. Problem solved!

When I made the soap, I omitted any scent. But if I made it again, I would use an ounce or more of fragrance per pound of fats, and I would choose something strong. Not a floral, not a sweet fragrance. Something woodsy or piney, or maybe musk, moss, amber, or sweetgrass. Just be careful to avoid scent that adds to the acceleration of the pine tar!

    7.2 oz (204 g) lard
    9 oz (255 g) coconut oil
    6 oz (170 g) almond oil
    6 oz (170 g) olive oil
    10.2 oz (289 g) water
    1 tbsp sugar
    4.2 oz (118 g) lye
    1.8 oz (51 g) creosote-free liquid pine tar

On the day before, dissolve the sugar in the water and freeze in cubes.

Pine tar is messy, so use disposable cups, spoons, and other utensils as much as you can. To minimize cleanup, I covered my work counter with newspaper.

For a mold, you'll need a silicone loaf pan. The pan may retain the pine tar smell, so don't count on using it later for other soaps. (I picked one up from a thrift store.) The soap mixture in this recipe is about a quart (about a liter), but the mold should be larger than that to allow stirring without spilling over.

Before you begin, put the mold on a tray or other flat, solid, movable surface. It's best if this "trivet" has a raised edge, in case the soap mixture does spill over.

Stick blend the soap mixture in the pot only till it thickens slightly, and pour into the mold. Then quickly add the pine tar and hand stir till well mixed, thoroughly working the pine tar into the corners and edges. By this time the soap will be quite thick, and you can leave it to set.

Designing Soaps with Accelerants

To keep things manageable, avoid combining accelerants. For instance, if you've chosen an accelerant that is a fat or additive, avoid also using an accelerating fragrance oil or essential oil. If your accelerant is a scent or additive, avoid accelerating fats like castor oil or shea oil. In fact, in this case, it's best to choose fats that are especially slow to saponify, like olive oil. Look for a low INS value as a likely sign of this.

Other additional accelerants you might want to avoid include sweeteners like honey, sugar, and fruit juice. On the other hand, they do boost lather, so they might sometimes be worth it.

If you don't know if something is an accelerant, search online. If other soapmakers have had trouble with it, you're sure to find something about it.

One way you can slow down saponification is by increasing liquid. For instance, my recipes normally include liquid in a percentage of 30% of the weight of the fats—but with an accelerant, I might increase this to 38%.

Keep volume down. The more soap you make at a time, the more heat is generated. This is true at all times, but with an accelerant in the mix, it's easy to generate too much.

A soap mixture with accelerant is probably not a good choice for swirling or another fancy color effect, since you won't have much time to work on it. Also, avoid fragile liquids like milk that don't tolerate higher temperatures.

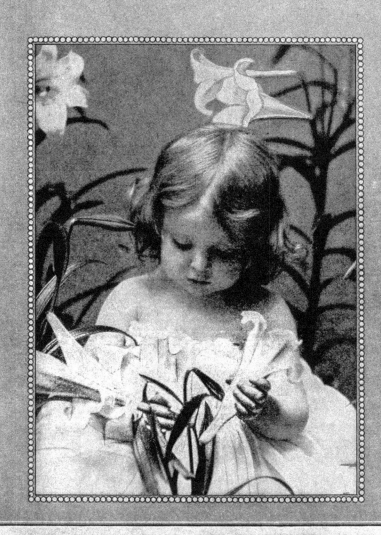

Ad for Packer's Tar Soap

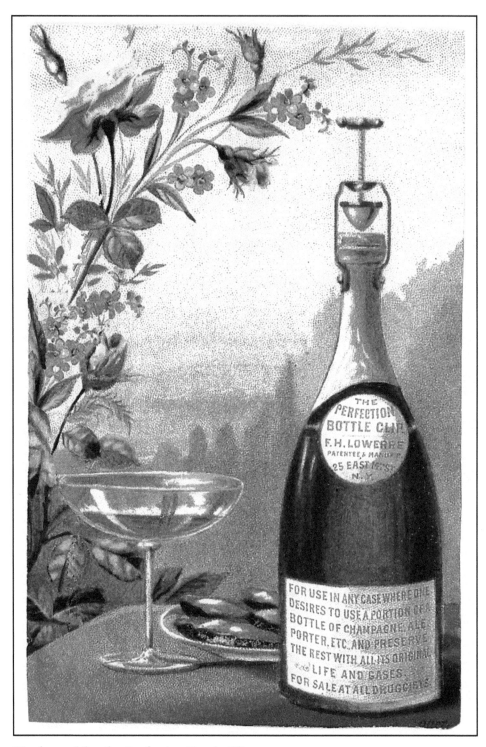

Trade card for the Perfection Bottle Clip

Project #5
Beer and Wine Soaps

As far as I can tell, the popularity of beer and wine soaps is a recent development. As fascinated as I am with antique soap advertisements, I've never run across one for a beer or wine soap.

I have to admit, I was less than enthusiastic when readers first asked me about soap made with beer or wine. I couldn't imagine washing with something that smelled like either one. Fortunately, it doesn't! And I discovered that the sugars and starches in these ingredients can make soap with excellent lather.

Soap made with beer or wine is prone to overheating, and it's easy to get a "volcano" or have the soap boil over in the mold. The usual way to deal with that is to trickle in the lye a few grains at a time—but Cool Technique makes that unnecessary.

Of course, beer and wine are not standardized products. Different varieties or even different brands may give you different results or require some adjustment in your methods. You'll need to experiment.

The beer in my own experiments was very ordinary supermarket beer—the kind you might be offered at a pizza restaurant or on a picnic. For wine, I used domestic cabernet sauvignon and chardonnay—the kind of wine a restaurant might serve in carafes. The alcohol content of both wines was 12%. I assumed that most soapmakers would be looking for inexpensive dry wine—not fine table wine, but not rotgut, either.

There are two factors in beer and wine soapmaking that you don't get with other kinds: carbonation and alcohol.

Carbonation doesn't work well with soapmaking, so you must flatten any beer or sparkling wine, whether or not you're using

Cool Technique. You could simply let it sit at room temperature till it's flat, but there's one problem: It's likely to mold. Even covered, it can pick up enough mold spores from somewhere—or maybe they're already in there—to develop some impressive fungi.

The quicker and better way is to add a pinch of baking powder, salt, sugar, cocoa, or almost any other granular substance that you're willing to have in your soap. Whip with a whisk to make it foam, and let the foam subside. If you repeat this several times, the beer or wine will go flat quickly. Using a wide bowl also helps, as it increases the surface area.

You can choose what to do about alcohol. I did not find it to be an accelerant. And though alcohol lowers the freezing temperature of the liquid, I didn't see any effect of this with beer. Wine may freeze unevenly, with the water content of the wine becoming more solid than the rest—but since I freeze in ice cube trays, I don't worry about that, either. I'll get the whole thing even if it separates somewhat.

Some soapmakers don't want alcohol in their soap because they find it drying. Again, I did not find this a problem—maybe because some of the alcohol evaporates during soapmaking. But I encourage you to experiment and see what you think.

I did find one drawback to the alcohol: It makes the lye dissolve more slowly. So, give that more time, and keep stirring gently. Be careful that *all* the lye is dissolved—this may be hard to tell, since the liquid will be dark and not completely transparent. When you pour the lye solution into the fats, pour through a sieve to make sure.

If you decide to get rid of the alcohol, you can do that by simmering the liquid for a couple of hours before weighing and freezing it. Or simply use commercial nonalcoholic beer or wine. Either way, you'll still get trace amounts of alcohol, but not enough to make a difference in soapmaking. You may also be able to get unfermented beer from home brewers, or unfermented wine from home winemakers. These will have neither alcohol nor carbonation.

If you're sensitive to the ammonia-like fumes of milk soapmaking, be aware you may get similar fumes with beer or wine. Handle this with increased ventilation.

Though beer and wine soap don't retain the odor of those liquids, they're not odorless, and the odor won't complement all fragrances. I avoid floral scents in favor of wood, musk, or herbal. Honey scent works well in beer soap. Of course, there are beer and wine fragrances too, if that's what you're aiming for.

Overall, I've preferred the beer soaps I've made to the wine ones. Though wine didn't hurt the soap, it was beer that really helped it. Beer soap, with all its sugar and starch, lathers particularly well.

Basic Beer Soap

9 oz (255 g) lard
4.5 oz (128 g) coconut oil
6 oz (171 g) grapeseed oil
10.5 oz (298 g) olive oil
9 oz (255 g) beer
2 tsp sugar
4.1 oz (116 g) lye
1.2–2 oz (34–56 g) essential oil or fragrance oil

The day before, combine the beer and sugar, stir to remove bubbles, and freeze in cubes.

Chocolate Ale Soap

15 oz (425 g) beef tallow
12 oz (340 g) palm kernel oil
3 oz (85 g) shea butter
1½ tbsp honey
9 oz (255 g) ale
1 tbsp cocoa powder
4.4 oz (125 g) lye
1.2–2 oz (34–56 g) essential oil or fragrance oil

The day before, combine the ale and cocoa powder and stir to remove bubbles. Add the honey and freeze in cubes.

Red Wine Soap

If you want red wine soap to be red, you will have to add colorant—the pigment in red wine does not stand up to saponification. The natural color of red wine soap is beige!

    15 oz (425 g) grapeseed oil
    6 oz (171 g) olive oil
    9 oz (255 g) coconut oil
    9 oz (255 g) red wine, frozen
    4.2 oz (118 g) lye

White Wine Soap

The fats in this soap were chosen for minimum color.

    9.9 oz (281 g) almond oil
    10.2 oz (289 g) avocado butter
    9.9 oz (281 g) coconut oil
    9 oz (255 g) white wine, frozen
    4.3 oz (123 g) lye

Anne's Coconut Beer Soap

This is the soap I'm now making for myself—my current favorite of all the recipes I've tried over the past couple of decades. It's 100% coconut oil soap made with beer as the liquid. I decided to try the duo because both beer and coconut oil produce rich lather.

The result is spectacular, with lather that's thick and rich, almost like whipped cream. One reservation is that I wouldn't use it for facial soap, since coconut oil can contribute to acne. But for bath and hand soap, it's in a class by itself.

Different beers will accelerate at different rates. So, depending on the particular beer you use, this recipe may need more or less special handling. For this reason, I don't recommend it for beginners. But it's worth the special care, in my opinion. The instructions given below represent what I would call the worst case, but you may have to experiment.

The superfatting for this 100% coconut oil soap is much higher than usual—20%. Don't add essential oils or fragrance oils that are accelerants themselves.

> 30 oz (851 g) coconut oil
> 9 oz (255 g) beer
> 2 tsp sugar
> 4.4 oz (125 g) lye
> 1.2–2 oz (34–56 g) essential oil or fragrance oil

The day before, combine the beer and sugar, stir to remove bubbles, and freeze in cubes.

Let the melted coconut oil cool to between 90°F and 100°F (32°C and 38°C) before adding the lye solution through a sieve.

Hand stir to mix. Don't use any kind of mechanical mixing—even a couple of bursts with a stick blender will be too much.

As you hand stir, the mixture will at first be transparent and honey-colored. Watch it carefully. As it starts to thicken, it will stay honey-colored but become more translucent. Let it thicken a little, to the consistency of warm honey. This is when you pour it into the mold. If it becomes opaque and white, it has gone too far.

I recommend a tray mold for this soap to keep it from overheating as it sets. If you use a log mold instead, refrigerate it after pouring. Keep checking the temperature of the outside of the mold with your hand. When the outside of the mold seems cool to your hand, you can remove the mold from the refrigerator, but keep checking after that. If you feel the mold heating up, cool it down again. If it overheats, the soap will develop a dark "bull's-eye" at the center.

Designing Beer and Wine Soaps

Since beer and wine are accelerants, avoid adding others, including accelerating fats like shea oil or castor oil.

When selecting wine or beer for soapmaking, be aware of the sugar and starch content. These carbohydrates contribute to both lather and acceleration. Beer has about one ounce of carbohydrates per quart (about 30 grams per liter). Light beers may have less; ales and specialty malt beverages may have more. The sugar content of wines varies from zero to about eight ounces per quart (about 220 grams per liter). Cheaper wines tend to have more sugar.

Also be aware of the alcohol content, which for commercial beverages will be noted on the label. More alcohol will mean slower dissolving for the lye. Beer is typically a little under 5% alcohol. Wine varies from about 6% to about 16%, with some wines considerably higher.

Color can be an important factor in the appeal of wine soap. Red wine by itself produces beige soap—so if that's not what you want, you will have to add colorant. White wine doesn't add its own color, but that might leave your soap with a tan color that again is not what you want. For a pale base color, use very pale fats like almond oil or coconut oil.

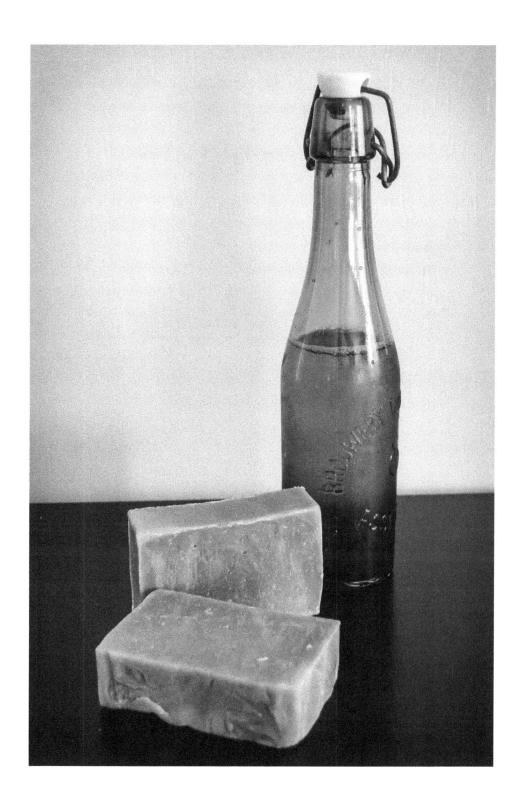

Why? Why? Why?
Frequently Asked Questions

How can I tell if a soap recipe is a good candidate for Cool Technique?

It's good to work low-temp if you have ingredients of the following kinds:

• Anything likely to scorch and discolor with heat, like milk.

• A fruit or vegetable that will smell bad after heating, like cucumber.

• A scent that will break down or dissipate if heated, like citrus.

• Anything—fat, liquid, scent, or additive—that will accelerate the chemical reaction or cause excessive heating.

• Anything that will produce strong fumes during soapmaking, like milk, beer, or wine.

Help! I got soda ash!

Soda ash—the soapmaker's name for a harmless but unsightly powdery residue that sometimes appears on the soap's surface—seems to be more common with Cool Technique. Generally, you can avoid it by spreading plastic wrap across the surface of the soap as it sets in the mold—but I don't know any completely reliable way to prevent it.

If you do wind up with it, you can at least take steps to get rid of it. The old advice was to rub the soap with alcohol. This does remove the residue, but it also makes the soap look used, making it unsuited for sale or gift-giving.

You can get surprisingly good results—at least with some soaps—by dunking the bar in water without rubbing it. But this might not work for soaps with detailed patterns on the surface—I imagine they'd blur and look used.

I've gotten my best results with steam, and I've bought a clothing steamer for the purpose. It's quite surprising how little steam is needed. A steam iron, though, might not do as well.

Help! My soap didn't harden!

If your soap starts to thicken and saponify but fails to set fully in the mold, put the mold somewhere warm—meaning about the temperature you'd use for bread dough or yogurt. Keep checking it. The soap might finish setting in a couple of hours, or it might take overnight or longer. Time and warmth should do it. It will also set more as you let it cool.

Author Online!

For updates, more resources, and
personal answers to your questions,
visit Anne's Soapmaking Page at

www.annelwatson.com/soapmaking

Where to Find More

Anne's Soapmaking Page

Check here for my latest experiments in soapmaking. There's always more to try and to learn!

www.annelwatson.com/soapmaking

SoapCalc

This site is one of the most useful sources of soapmaking information and formula analysis. It's nearly indispensable for designing your own recipes.

www.soapcalc.net

About the Author

Anne L. Watson is the first author to have introduced modern techniques of home soapmaking and lotionmaking to book readers. She has made soap under the company name Soap Tree, and before her retirement from professional life, she was a historic preservation architecture consultant.

Besides her soap and lotion books, Anne has written practical guides to such topics as cookie molds and housekeeping, along with a number of literary novels. She and her husband, Aaron Shepard, live in Bellingham, Washington. You can visit her at

www.annelwatson.com

Lightning Source UK Ltd.
Milton Keynes UK
UKHW020728291219
355991UK00003B/41/P